4 Week Meal Plan for Weight Loss

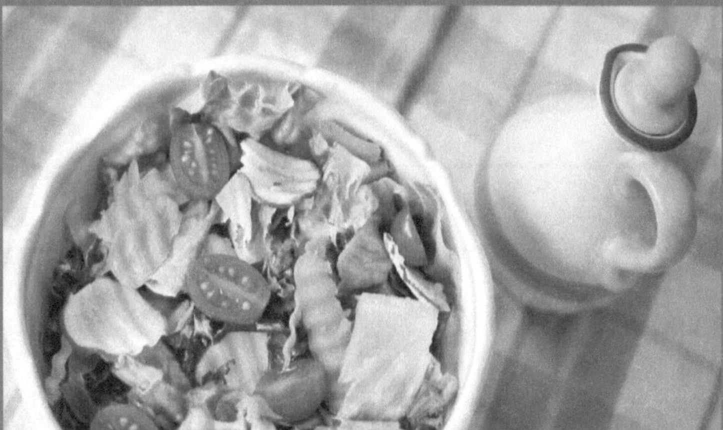

TABLE OF CONTENTS

MEALS IN THIS PLAN

BREAKFAST:

- ✓ Greek yogurt with mixed berries and granola
- ✓ Scrambled eggs with spinach and whole wheat toast
- ✓ Overnight oats with almond milk, sliced banana, and chia seeds
- ✓ Protein smoothie with mixed berries, spinach, and almond milk
- ✓ Whole grain waffles with sliced strawberries and a drizzle of maple syrup

SNACKS:

- ✓ Apple with almond butter
- ✓ Banana with a handful of almonds
- ✓ Baby carrots with hummus
- ✓ Baby carrots with ranch dressing
- ✓ Boiled egg with whole grain crackers
- ✓ Pear with cheese
- ✓ Small handful of cashews
- ✓ Greek yogurt with sliced peaches

LUNCH:

- ✓ Grilled chicken salad with mixed greens, cherry tomatoes, cucumber, and a vinaigrette dressing
- ✓ Tuna salad with mixed greens and whole wheat crackers
- ✓ Turkey and avocado wrap with a side salad
- ✓ Grilled shrimp salad with mixed greens, cherry tomatoes, cucumber, and a vinaigrette dressing
- ✓ Grilled chicken with sweet potato and roasted vegetables

DINNER:

- ✓ Grilled salmon with roasted asparagus and quinoa

- ✓ Spaghetti squash with turkey meatballs and marinara sauce

- ✓ Beef stir-fry with brown rice and mixed vegetables

- ✓ Baked chicken with roasted Brussels sprouts and brown rice

- ✓ Grilled fish with a side of roasted vegetables and quinoa

4 WEEK MEAL PLAN FOR WEIGHT LOSS

Week 1:

Monday

Breakfast: Greek yogurt with mixed berries and a sprinkle of granola

Snack: An apple with almond butter

Lunch: Grilled chicken salad with mixed greens, cherry tomatoes, cucumber, and a vinaigrette dressing

Snack: Carrot sticks with hummus

Dinner: Grilled salmon with roasted asparagus and quinoa

Tuesday

Breakfast: Scrambled eggs with spinach and whole wheat toast

Snack: A banana with a handful of almonds

Lunch: Turkey and avocado wrap with a side salad

Snack: Greek yogurt with sliced peaches

Dinner: Spaghetti squash with turkey meatballs and marinara sauce

Wednesday

Breakfast: Overnight oats with almond milk, sliced banana, and chia seeds

Snack: Baby carrots with ranch dressing

Lunch: Grilled chicken with sweet potato and roasted vegetables

Snack: A pear with cheese

Dinner: Beef stir-fry with brown rice and mixed vegetables

Thursday

Breakfast: Protein smoothie with mixed berries, spinach, and almond milk

Snack: A boiled egg with whole grain crackers

Lunch: Grilled shrimp salad with mixed greens, cherry tomatoes, cucumber, and a vinaigrette dressing

Snack: A small handful of cashews

Dinner: Baked chicken with roasted Brussels sprouts and brown rice

Friday

Breakfast: Whole grain waffles with sliced strawberries and a drizzle of maple syrup

Snack: Baby carrots with hummus

Lunch: Tuna salad with mixed greens and whole wheat crackers

Snack: A peach with cottage cheese

Dinner: Grilled fish with a side of roasted vegetables and quinoa

Saturday/Sunday

Pick a recipe from the list on pages 2 and 3 for each meal of the day to mix it up and enjoy the food you choose for the weekend. Back to the plan on Monday!

Week 2:

Monday

Breakfast: Scrambled eggs with spinach and whole wheat toast

Snack: A pear with cheese

Lunch: Tuna salad with mixed greens and whole wheat crackers

Snack: Baby carrots with hummus

Dinner: Grilled fish with a side of roasted vegetables and quinoa

Tuesday

Breakfast: Greek yogurt with mixed berries and a sprinkle of granola

Snack: A small handful of cashews

Lunch: Grilled shrimp salad with mixed greens, cherry tomatoes, cucumber, and a vinaigrette dressing

Snack: A boiled egg with whole grain crackers

Dinner: Baked chicken with roasted Brussels sprouts and brown rice

Wednesday

Breakfast: Whole grain waffles with sliced strawberries and a drizzle of maple syrup

Snack: Baby carrots with ranch dressing

Lunch: Grilled chicken with sweet potato and roasted vegetables

Snack: A peach with cottage cheese

Dinner: Beef stir-fry with brown rice and mixed vegetables

Thursday

Breakfast: Overnight oats with almond milk, sliced banana, and chia seeds

Snack: An apple with almond butter

Lunch: Grilled chicken salad with mixed greens, cherry tomatoes, cucumber, and a vinaigrette dressing

Snack: Greek yogurt with sliced peaches

Dinner: Spaghetti squash with turkey meatballs and marinara sauce

Friday

Breakfast: Protein smoothie with mixed berries, spinach, and almond milk

Snack: Baby carrots with hummus

Lunch: Turkey and avocado wrap with a side salad

Snack: A banana with a handful of almonds

Dinner: Grilled salmon with roasted asparagus and quinoa

Saturday/Sunday

Pick a recipe from the list on pages 2 and 3 for each meal of the day to mix it up and enjoy the food you choose for the weekend. Back to the plan on Monday!

Week 3:

Monday

Breakfast: Greek yogurt with mixed berries and a sprinkle of granola

Snack: An apple with almond butter

Lunch: Grilled chicken salad with mixed greens, cherry tomatoes, cucumber, and a vinaigrette dressing

Snack: Carrot sticks with hummus

Dinner: Grilled salmon with roasted asparagus and quinoa

Tuesday

Breakfast: Scrambled eggs with spinach and whole wheat toast

Snack: A banana with a handful of almonds

Lunch: Turkey and avocado wrap with a side salad

Snack: Greek yogurt with sliced peaches

Dinner: Spaghetti squash with turkey meatballs and marinara sauce

Wednesday

Breakfast: Overnight oats with almond milk, sliced banana, and chia seeds

Snack: Baby carrots with ranch dressing

Lunch: Grilled chicken with sweet potato and roasted vegetables

Snack: A pear with cheese

Dinner: Beef stir-fry with brown rice and mixed vegetables

Thursday

Breakfast: Protein smoothie with mixed berries, spinach, and almond milk

Snack: A boiled egg with whole grain crackers

Lunch: Grilled shrimp salad with mixed greens, cherry tomatoes, cucumber, and a vinaigrette dressing

Snack: A small handful of cashews

Dinner: Baked chicken with roasted Brussels sprouts and brown rice

Friday

Breakfast: Overnight oats with almond milk, sliced banana, and chia seeds

Snack: A banana with a handful of almonds

Lunch: Grilled chicken salad with mixed greens, cherry tomatoes, cucumber, and a vinaigrette dressing

Snack: Greek yogurt with sliced peaches

Dinner: Spaghetti squash with turkey meatballs and marinara sauce

Saturday/Sunday

Pick a recipe from the list on pages 2 and 3 for each meal of the day to mix it up and enjoy the food you choose for the weekend. Back to the plan on Monday!

Week 4:

Monday

Breakfast: Whole grain waffles with sliced strawberries and a drizzle of maple syrup

Snack: Baby carrots with hummus

Lunch: Grilled chicken with sweet potato and roasted vegetables

Snack: A peach with cottage cheese

Dinner: Beef stir-fry with brown rice and mixed vegetables

Tuesday

Breakfast: Protein smoothie with mixed berries, spinach, and almond milk

Snack: Baby carrots with ranch dressing

Lunch: Tuna salad with mixed greens and whole wheat crackers

Snack: A small handful of cashews

Dinner: Grilled fish with a side of roasted vegetables and quinoa

Wednesday

Breakfast: Scrambled eggs with spinach and whole wheat toast

Snack: A boiled egg with whole grain crackers

Lunch: Grilled shrimp salad with mixed greens, cherry tomatoes, cucumber, and a vinaigrette dressing

Snack: A pear with cheese

Dinner: Baked chicken with roasted Brussels sprouts and brown rice

Thursday

Breakfast: Greek yogurt with mixed berries and a sprinkle of granola

Snack: An apple with almond butter

Lunch: Turkey and avocado wrap with a side salad

Snack: Greek yogurt with sliced peaches

Dinner: Spaghetti squash with turkey meatballs and marinara sauce

Friday

Breakfast: Overnight oats with almond milk, sliced banana, and chia seeds

Snack: A banana with a handful of almonds

Lunch: Grilled chicken salad with mixed greens, cherry tomatoes, cucumber, and a vinaigrette dressing

Snack: Greek yogurt with sliced peaches

Dinner: Spaghetti squash with turkey meatballs and marinara sauce

Saturday/Sunday

Pick a recipe from the list on pages 2 and 3 for each meal of the day to mix it up and enjoy the food you choose for the weekend. Back to the plan on Monday!

BREAKFAST

Greek Yogurt with Mixed Berries and Granola:

Ingredients:

1 cup plain Greek yogurt

1/2 cup mixed berries (such as blueberries, raspberries, and strawberries)

1/4 cup granola

Directions:

✓ Wash and dry the mixed berries.

✓ In a bowl, mix together the Greek yogurt and mixed berries.

Top with granola, and enjoy!

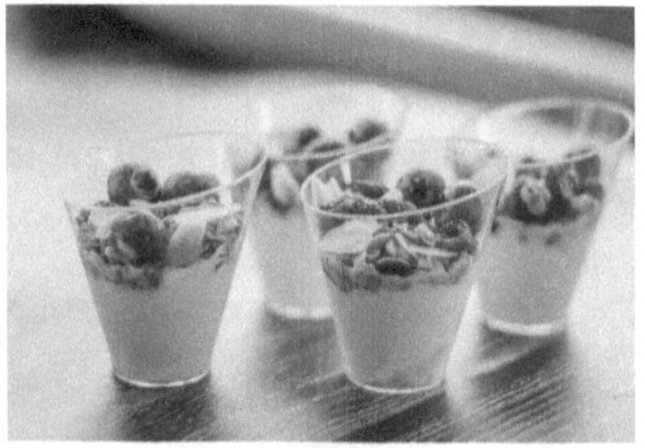

Scrambled Eggs with Spinach and Whole Wheat Toast

Ingredients:

2 eggs

1/4 cup spinach, chopped

1 slice of whole wheat bread

Salt and pepper to taste

1 tsp olive oil

Directions:

✓ Beat the eggs in a small bowl, and season with salt and pepper.

✓ Heat the olive oil in a small skillet over medium heat.

✓ Add the chopped spinach to the skillet and cook until wilted.

✓ Pour the beaten eggs over the spinach and stir gently until scrambled and cooked through.

✓ Toast the slice of whole wheat bread.

Serve the scrambled eggs with the whole wheat toast on the side.

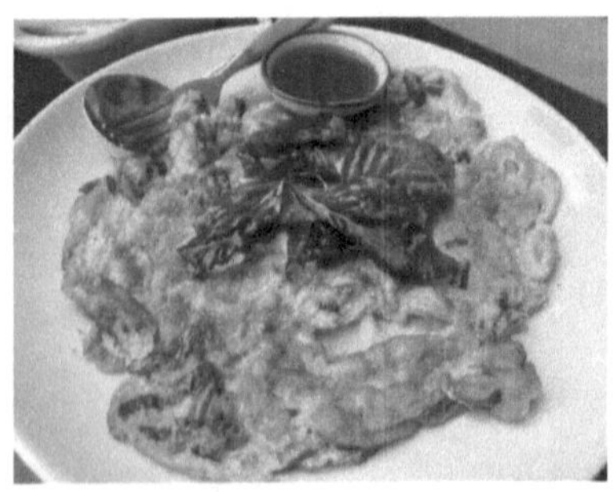

Overnight Oats with Almond Milk, Sliced Banana, and Chia Seeds

Ingredients:

1/2 cup rolled oats

1/2 cup unsweetened almond milk

1/2 banana, sliced

1 tbsp chia seeds

1 tbsp honey (optional)

Directions:

✓ In a small jar or container, mix together the rolled oats, almond milk, chia seeds, and honey (if using).

✓ Cover the container and refrigerate overnight.

In the morning, top with sliced banana, and enjoy!

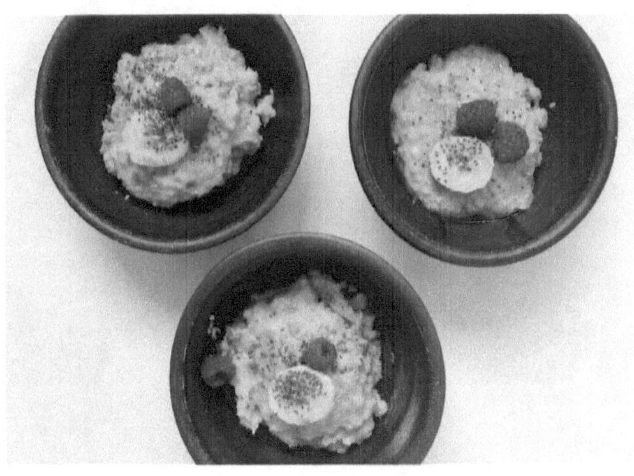

Protein Smoothie with Mixed Berries, Spinach, and Almond Milk

Ingredients:

1 cup mixed berries (such as blueberries, raspberries, and strawberries)

1 cup spinach

1 scoop protein powder

1 cup unsweetened almond milk

Directions:

- ✓ Wash and dry the mixed berries and spinach.

- ✓ In a blender, blend together the mixed berries, spinach, protein powder, and almond milk until smooth.

Pour into a glass and enjoy!

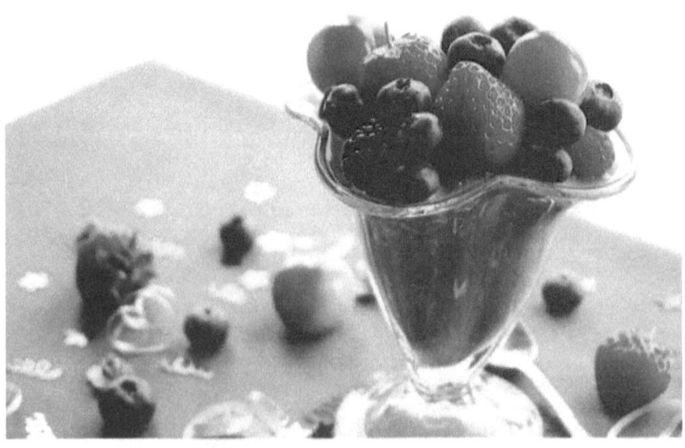

Whole Grain Waffles with Sliced Strawberries and a Drizzle of Maple Syrup

Ingredients:

2 whole grain waffles

1/2 cup sliced strawberries

1 tbsp maple syrup

Directions:

✓ Toast the whole grain waffles in a toaster or toaster oven.

✓ Top with sliced strawberries and drizzle with maple syrup. Enjoy!

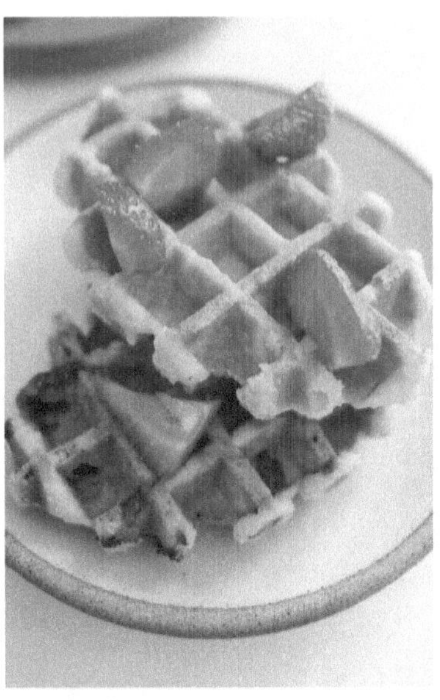

SNACKS

Apple with Almond Butter

Ingredients:

1 apple, sliced

2 tbsp almond butter

Directions:

- ✓ Slice the apple into bite-sized pieces.

- ✓ Dip the apple slices into the almond butter, and enjoy!

Banana with a Handful of Almonds

Ingredients:

1 banana

Handful of almonds

Directions:

- ✓ Peel the banana and slice it into bite-sized pieces.

- ✓ Enjoy the banana with a handful of almonds.

Baby Carrots with Hummus

Ingredients:

1 cup baby carrots

1/4 cup hummus

Directions:

- ✓ Wash and dry the baby carrots.

- ✓ Serve the carrots with a side of hummus for dipping.

Baby Carrots with Ranch Dressing

Ingredients:

1 cup baby carrots

1/4 cup ranch dressing

Directions:

- ✓ Wash and dry the baby carrots.

- ✓ Serve the carrots with a side of ranch dressing for dipping.

Boiled Egg with Whole Grain Crackers

Ingredients:

1 boiled egg

Whole grain crackers

Directions:

- ✓ Peel the boiled egg and slice it in half.

- ✓ Serve the boiled egg with a side of whole grain crackers.

Pear with Cheese:

Ingredients:

1 pear, sliced

1 oz cheese

Directions:

- ✓ Slice the pear into bite-sized pieces.

- ✓ Serve the pear with a side of cheese

Greek Yogurt with Sliced Peaches

Ingredients:

1 cup plain Greek yogurt

1 peach, sliced

Directions:

- ✓ Wash and slice the peach into bite-sized pieces.

- ✓ Serve the Greek yogurt with a side of sliced peaches.

LUNCH

Grilled Chicken Salad with Mixed Greens, Cherry Tomatoes, Cucumber, and a Vinaigrette Dressing

Ingredients:

2 boneless, skinless chicken breasts

6 cups mixed greens

1 cup cherry tomatoes, halved

1/2 cup sliced cucumber

1/4 cup chopped red onion

2 tbsp olive oil

2 tbsp red wine vinegar

1 tsp Dijon mustard

Salt and pepper to taste

Directions:

- ✓ Preheat a grill or grill pan to medium-high heat.

- ✓ Season the chicken breasts with salt and pepper, and grill for 4-5 minutes on each side, or until cooked through.

- ✓ Let the chicken rest for a few minutes, then slice into strips.

- ✓ In a large bowl, whisk together the olive oil, red wine vinegar, Dijon mustard, salt, and pepper to make the vinaigrette.

✓ Add the mixed greens, cherry tomatoes, cucumber, and red onion to the bowl, and toss to coat with the vinaigrette.

Divide the salad between plates and top each plate with sliced grilled chicken.

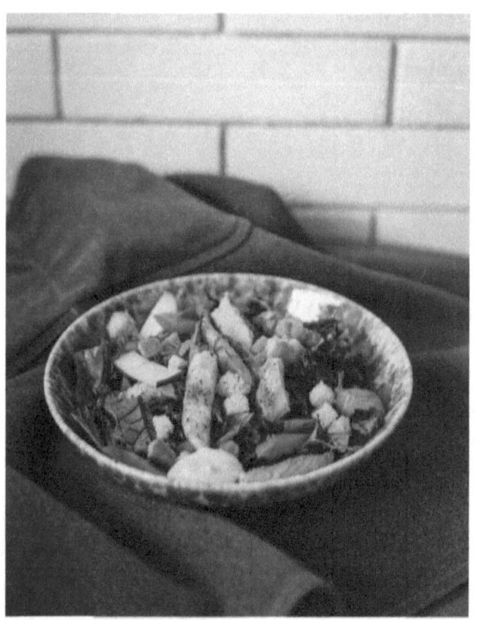

Tuna Salad with Mixed Greens and Whole Wheat Crackers

Ingredients:

2 (5 oz) cans of tuna, drained

1/4 cup chopped celery

1/4 cup chopped red onion

2 tbsp chopped fresh parsley

2 tbsp plain Greek yogurt

2 tbsp mayonnaise

1 tbsp Dijon mustard

Salt and pepper to taste

6 cups mixed greens

Whole wheat crackers for serving

Directions:

- ✓ In a medium-sized bowl, mix together the tuna, celery, red onion, parsley, Greek yogurt, mayonnaise, Dijon mustard, salt, and pepper.

- ✓ In a separate large bowl, toss the mixed greens with a drizzle of olive oil and a sprinkle of salt and pepper.

- ✓ Divide the mixed greens between plates and top each plate with a scoop of tuna salad.

Serve with whole wheat crackers on the side.

Turkey and Avocado Wrap with a Side Salad

Ingredients:

4 whole wheat tortillas

1 lb sliced turkey

1 avocado, sliced

1 cup shredded lettuce

1/2 cup sliced cherry tomatoes

2 tbsp plain Greek yogurt

1 tbsp lime juice

Salt and pepper to taste

Directions:

- ✓ In a small bowl, whisk together the Greek yogurt, lime juice, salt, and pepper to make a dressing for the side salad.
- ✓ In a large bowl, toss together the shredded lettuce and sliced cherry tomatoes with the dressing.
- ✓ Lay out the tortillas and divide the sliced turkey and sliced avocado between them.
- ✓ Roll up the tortillas, and slice in half.

Serve the turkey and avocado wraps with a side of the salad.

Grilled Shrimp Salad with Mixed Greens, Cherry Tomatoes, Cucumber, and a Vinaigrette Dressing

Ingredients:

1 lb shrimp, peeled and deveined

6 cups mixed greens

1 cup cherry tomatoes, halved

1/2 cup sliced cucumber

1/4 cup chopped red onion

2 tbsp olive oil

2 tbsp red wine vinegar

1 tsp Dijon mustard

Salt and pepper to taste

Directions:

Preheat a grill or grill pan to medium-high heat.

Season the shrimp with salt and pepper, and grill for 2-3 minutes on each side, or until cooked through.

In a large bowl, whisk together the olive oil, red wine vinegar, Dijon mustard, salt, and pepper to make the vinaigrette.

Add the mixed greens, cherry tomatoes, cucumber, and red onion to the bowl, and toss to coat with the vinaigrette.

Divide the salad between plates, and top each plate with grilled shrimp.

Grilled Chicken with Sweet Potato and Roasted Vegetables

Ingredients:

4 boneless, skinless chicken breasts

2 sweet potatoes, peeled and chopped into bite-sized pieces

2 cups mixed vegetables (such as zucchini, red bell pepper, and eggplant), sliced into bite-sized pieces

2 tbsp olive oil

1 tsp garlic powder

1 tsp paprika

Salt and pepper to taste

Directions:

Preheat the oven to 375°F.

Season the chicken breasts with salt, pepper, garlic powder, and paprika.

Heat a drizzle of oil in a grill pan or large skillet over medium-high heat.

Add the chicken breasts and cook for 4-5 minutes on each side, or until cooked through.

Remove the chicken from the pan and let it rest.

Meanwhile, in a large bowl, toss together the chopped sweet potatoes and mixed vegetables with olive oil, salt, and pepper.

Spread the vegetables in a single layer on a baking sheet.

Roast in the preheated oven for 20-25 minutes, or until the vegetables are tender and slightly browned.

Serve the grilled chicken with a side of roasted vegetables. Enjoy!

DINNER

Grilled Salmon With Roasted Asparagus And Quinoa

Ingredients:

4 (4 oz) salmon fillets

1 tbsp olive oil

Salt and pepper to taste

1 bunch asparagus, trimmed

1 cup quinoa

2 cups water

Directions:

✓ Preheat the grill to medium-high heat.

✓ Rinse and drain the quinoa. In a medium-sized saucepan, bring the quinoa and water to a boil. Reduce heat to low, cover, and simmer for 15-20 minutes or until the quinoa is tender and the water has been absorbed. Set aside.

✓ Place the asparagus in a single layer on a baking sheet. Drizzle with 1 tablespoon of olive oil and sprinkle with salt and pepper.

✓ Place the salmon fillets skin-side down on the grill, and season with salt and pepper. Grill for 4-5 minutes on each side, or until cooked through.

✓ Place the baking sheet with the asparagus in the oven and roast for 8-10 minutes, or until tender and slightly browned.

To serve, place a scoop of quinoa on each plate, top with a salmon fillet, and a few asparagus spears.

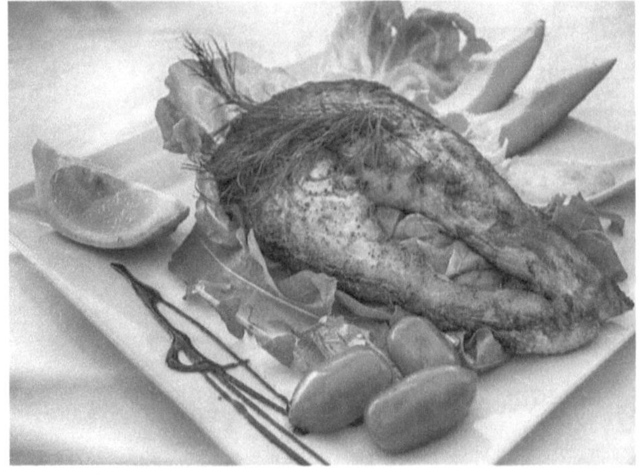

Spaghetti Squash With Turkey Meatballs And Marinara Sauce

Ingredients:

1 medium spaghetti squash

1 lb ground turkey

1/2 cup breadcrumbs

1 egg

1/4 cup grated Parmesan cheese

1/4 cup chopped fresh parsley

1/4 cup chopped fresh basil

1/4 cup chopped onion

2 cloves garlic, minced

Salt and pepper to taste

2 cups marinara sauce

Directions:

✓ Preheat the oven to 375°F.

✓ Cut the spaghetti squash in half lengthwise and remove the seeds with a spoon.

✓ Place the spaghetti squash halves cut-side down on a baking sheet, and bake for 40-45 minutes, or until the squash is tender.

✓ While the squash is baking, mix together the ground turkey, breadcrumbs, egg, Parmesan cheese, parsley, basil, onion, garlic, salt, and pepper in a large bowl.

- ✓ Roll the turkey mixture into meatballs, about 1-2 inches in diameter.
- ✓ In a large skillet, heat a drizzle of olive oil over medium heat. Add the meatballs and cook until browned on all sides.

- ✓ Pour the marinara sauce over the meatballs and let simmer for 10-15 minutes, until the meatballs are cooked through and the sauce has thickened slightly.

- ✓ Once the spaghetti squash is done baking, use a fork to scrape the squash flesh into long strands.

Serve the spaghetti squash topped with the turkey meatballs and marinara sauce.

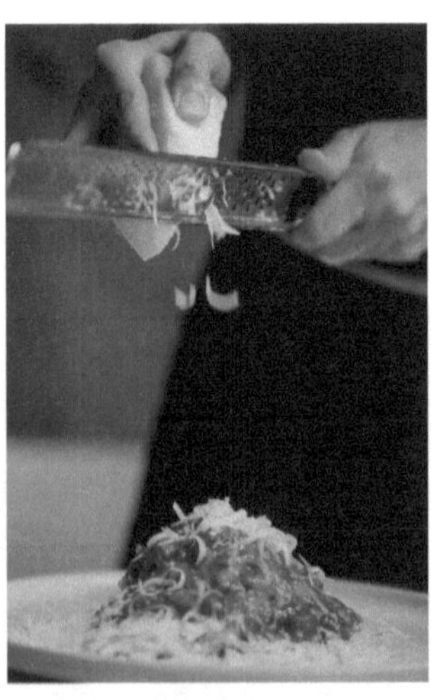

Beef Stir-Fry with Brown Rice and Mixed Vegetables

Ingredients:

1 lb flank steak, sliced thinly against the grain

2 tbsp cornstarch

2 tbsp soy sauce

1 tbsp sesame oil

2 cloves garlic, minced

1 inch ginger, grated

1 red bell pepper, sliced thinly

1 cup sliced mushrooms

2 cups mixed vegetables (broccoli, snap peas, carrots, etc.)

2 cups cooked brown ric1 lb flank steak, sliced thinly against the grain

2 tbsp cornstarch

2 tbsp soy sauce

1 tbsp sesame oil

2 cloves garlic, minced

1 inch ginger, grated

1 red bell pepper, sliced thinly

1 cup sliced mushrooms

2 cups mixed vegetables (broccoli, snap peas, carrots, etc.)

4 (4 oz) fish fillets (such as salmon, tilapia, or cod)

1 tbsp olive oil

1 tbsp lemon juice

1 clove garlic, minced

Salt and pepper to taste

2 cups mixed vegetables (such as zucchini, red bell pepper, and eggplant), sliced into bite-sized pieces

1 cup quinoa

2 cups water

Directions:

- ✓ In a large bowl, mix together the sliced beef, cornstarch, soy sauce, and sesame oil. Set aside.

- ✓ In a wok or large skillet, heat a drizzle of oil over high heat.

- ✓ Add the minced garlic and grated ginger, and stir-fry for 1 minute.

- ✓ Add the sliced bell pepper, mushrooms, and mixed vegetables, and stir-fry for 2-3 minutes, or until the vegetables are crisp-tender.

- ✓ Remove the vegetables from the wok and set aside.

- ✓ Add the beef to the wok and stir-fry for 2-3 minutes, or until browned and cooked through.

- ✓ Add the vegetables back to the wok and stir-fry for an additional minute.

Serve the beef stir-fry over cooked brown rice.

Baked Chicken with Roasted Brussels Sprouts and Brown Rice

Ingredients:

4 boneless, skinless chicken breasts

2 tbsp olive oil

1 tsp garlic powder

1 tsp paprika

Salt and pepper to taste

1 lb Brussels sprouts, trimmed and halved

2 cups cooked brown rice

Directions:

- ✓ Preheat the oven to 375°F.

- ✓ Place the chicken breasts in a baking dish.

- ✓ Drizzle the chicken with olive oil, and season with garlic powder, paprika, salt, and pepper.

- ✓ Arrange the Brussels sprouts around the chicken in the baking dish.

- ✓ Drizzle the Brussels sprouts with olive oil, and season with salt and pepper.

- ✓ Bake for 25-30 minutes, or until the chicken is cooked through and the Brussels sprouts are tender and slightly browned.

Serve the baked chicken and brussels sprouts over cooked brown rice.

Grilled Fish With A Side Of Roasted Vegetables And Quinoa

Ingredients:

4 (4 oz) fish fillets (such as salmon, tilapia, or cod)

1 tbsp olive oil

1 tbsp lemon juice

1 clove garlic, minced

Salt and pepper to taste

2 cups mixed vegetables (such as zucchini, red bell pepper, and eggplant), sliced into bite-sized pieces

1 cup quinoa

2 cups water

Directions:

- ✓ Rinse and drain the quinoa. In a medium-sized saucepan, bring the quinoa and water to a boil. Reduce heat to low, cover, and simmer for 15-20 minutes or until the quinoa is tender and the water has been absorbed. Set aside.

- ✓ Preheat the grill to medium-high heat.

- ✓ In a small bowl, whisk together the olive oil, lemon juice, minced garlic, salt, and pepper.

- ✓ Brush the fish fillets with the olive oil mixture.

- ✓ Place the fish fillets on the grill, and cook for 4-5 minutes on each side, or until cooked through.

✓ While the fish is cooking, spread the mixed vegetables in a single layer on a baking sheet. Drizzle with a little olive oil and season with salt and pepper.

✓ Place the baking sheet with the mixed vegetables in the oven and roast for 12-15 minutes, or until tender and slightly browned.

To serve, place a scoop of quinoa on each plate, top with a grilled fish fillet, and a side of roasted mixed vegetables. Enjoy!

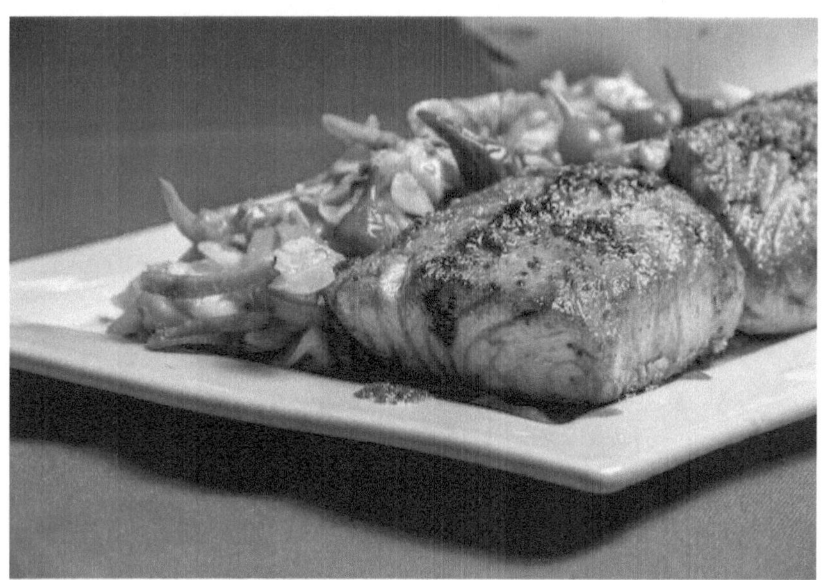